Coloring book

I

AM

A

DOCTOR

Coloring book

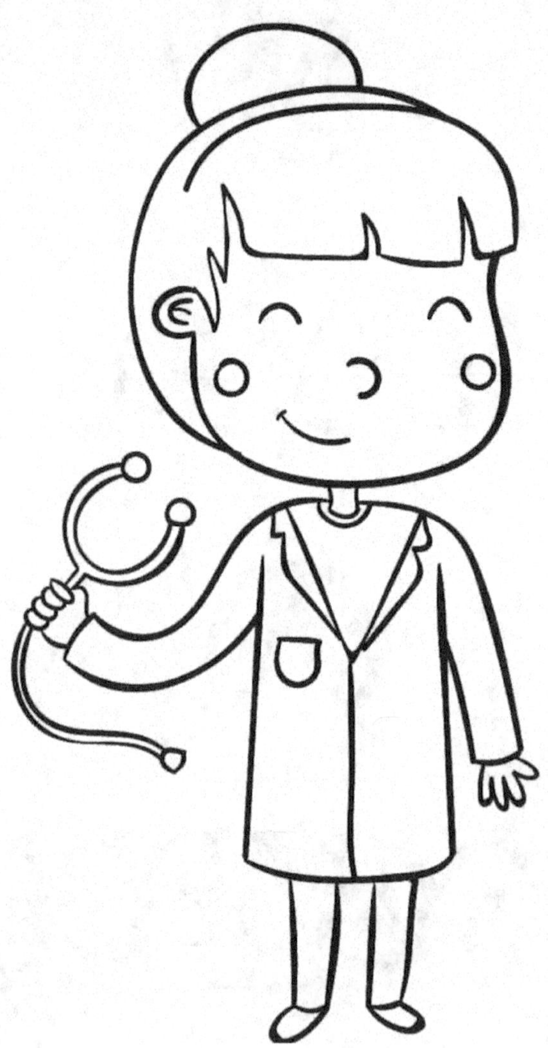

Coloring book

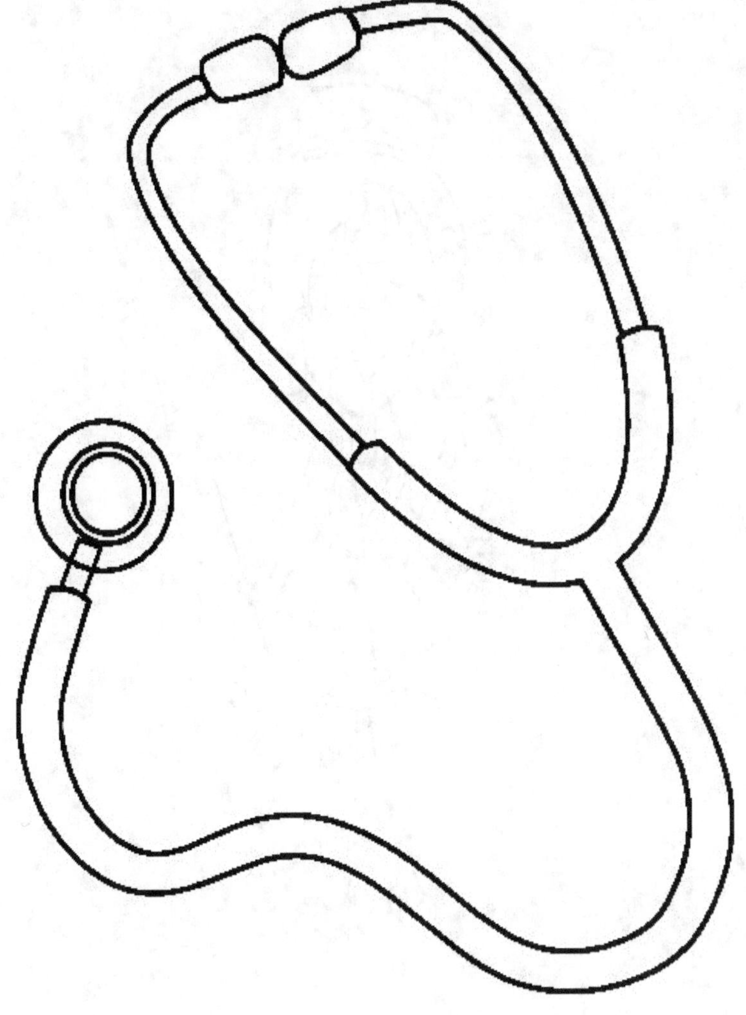

Coloring book

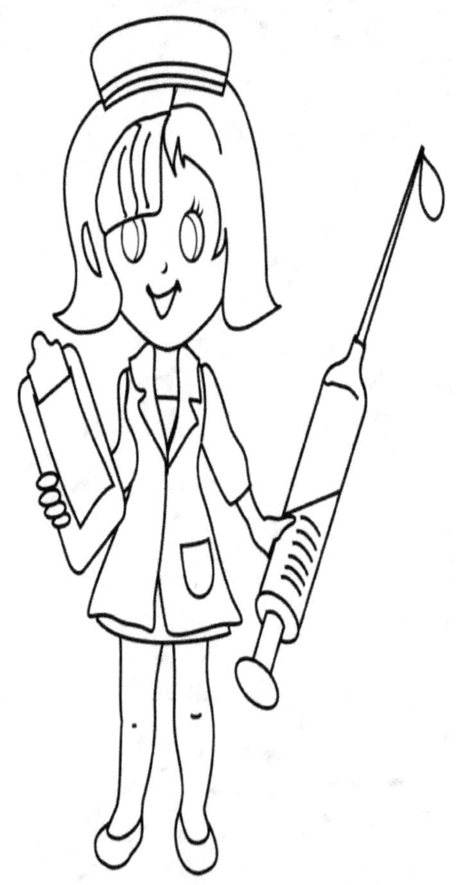

Coloring book

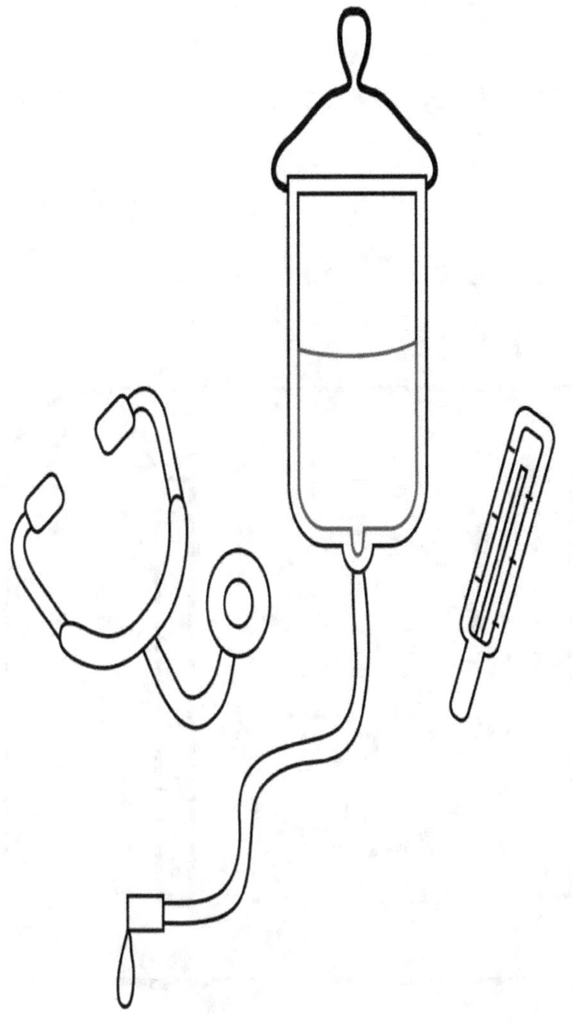

Coloring book

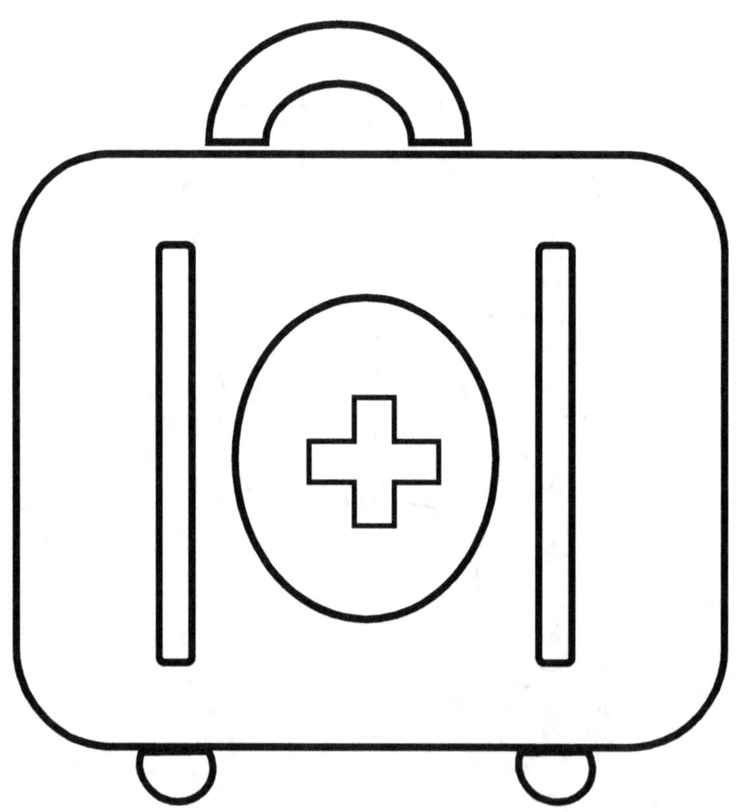

Coloring book

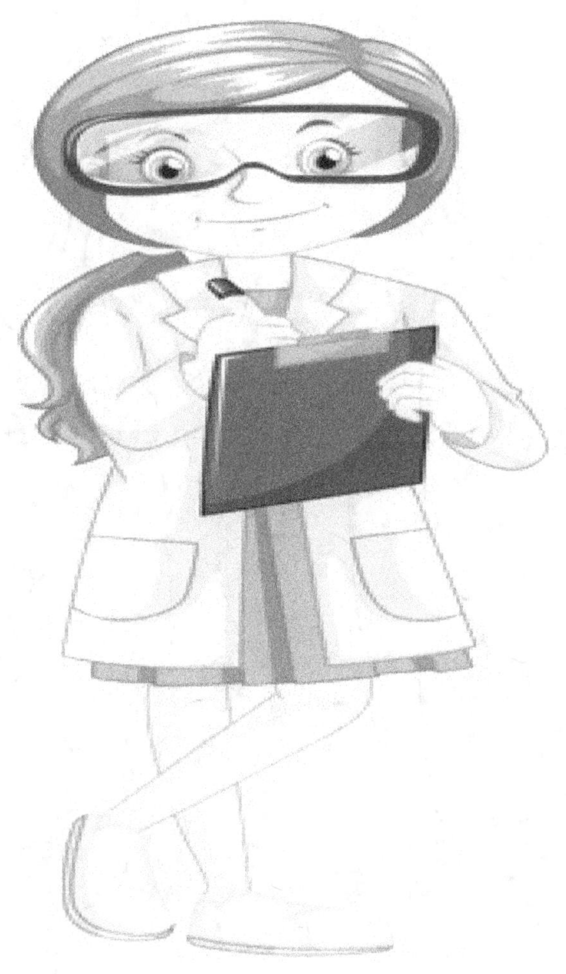

Coloring book

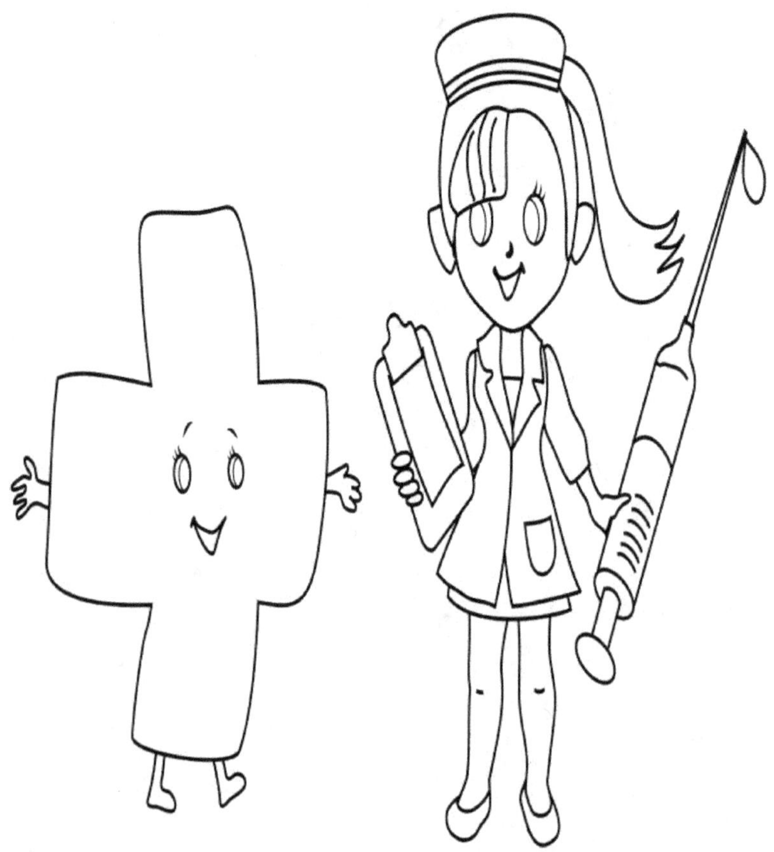

Coloring book

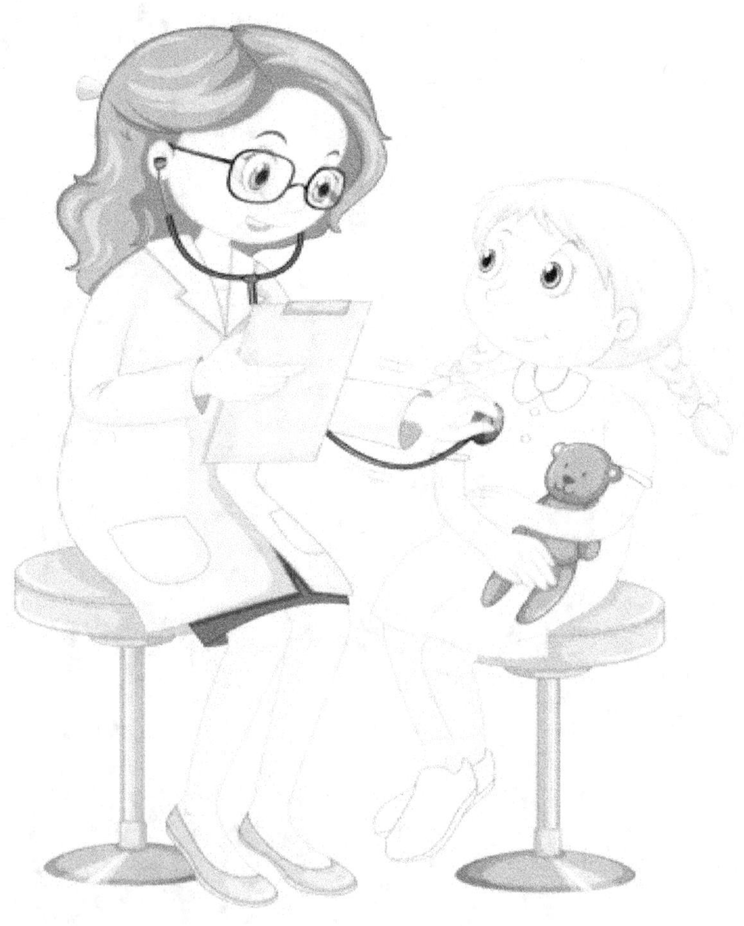

Coloring book

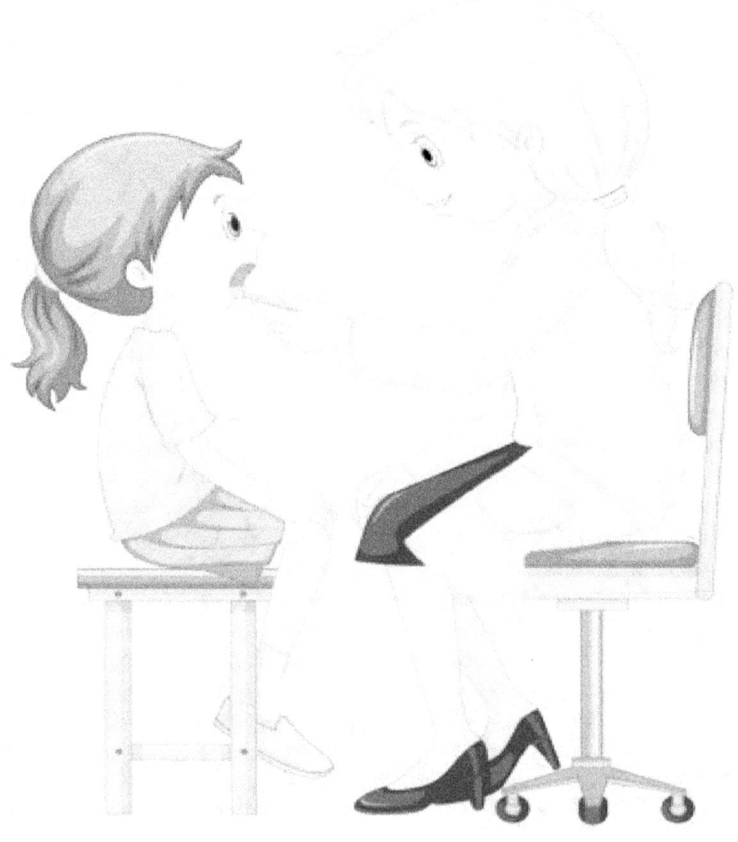

Coloring book

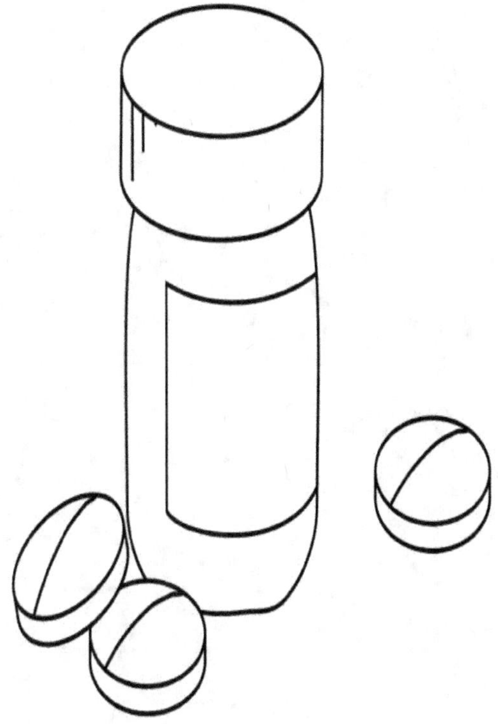

Coloring book

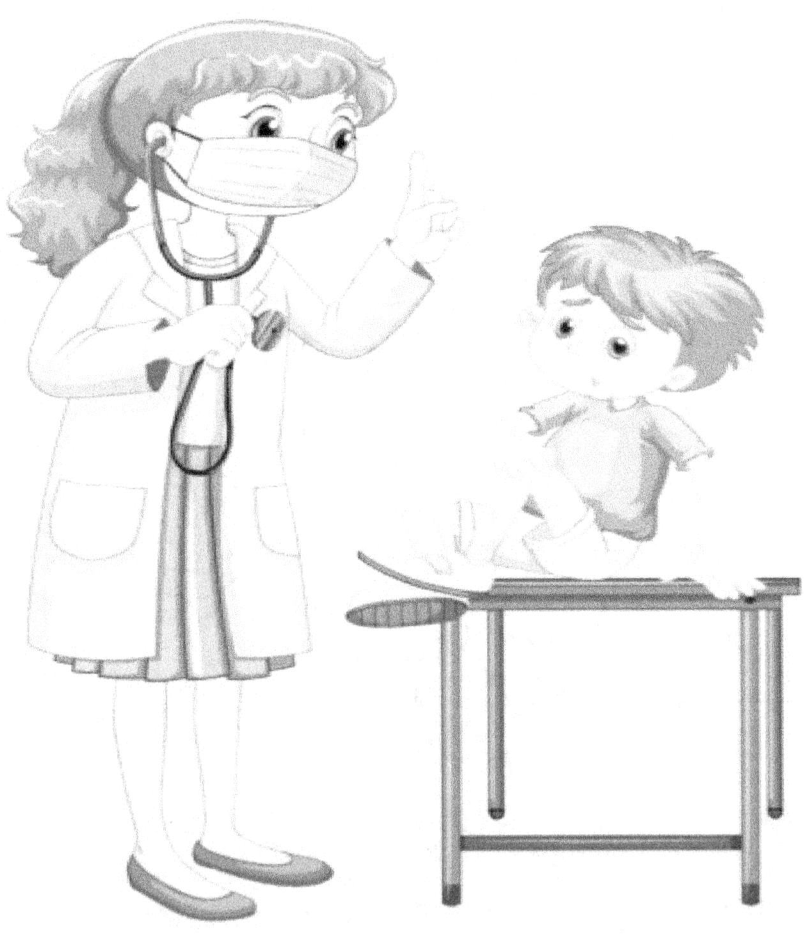

Coloring book

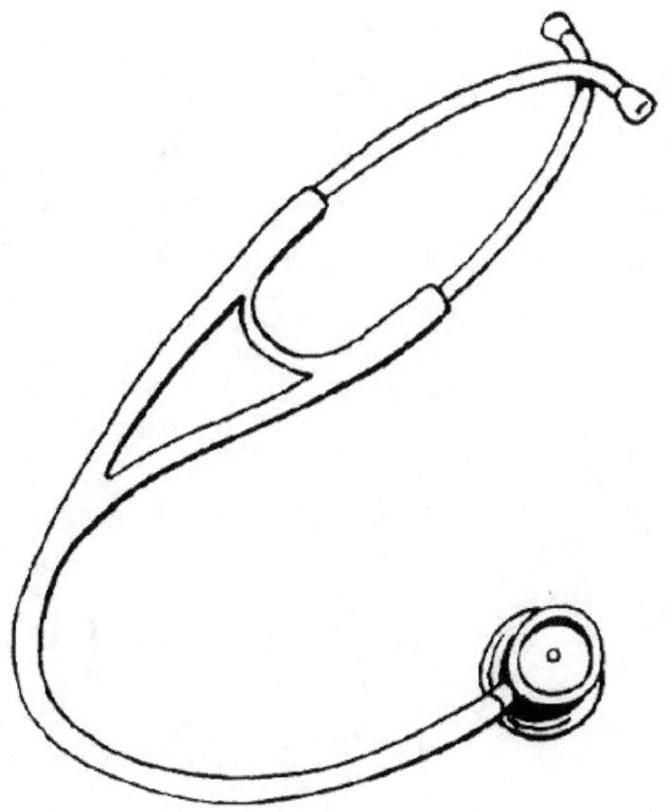

Coloring book

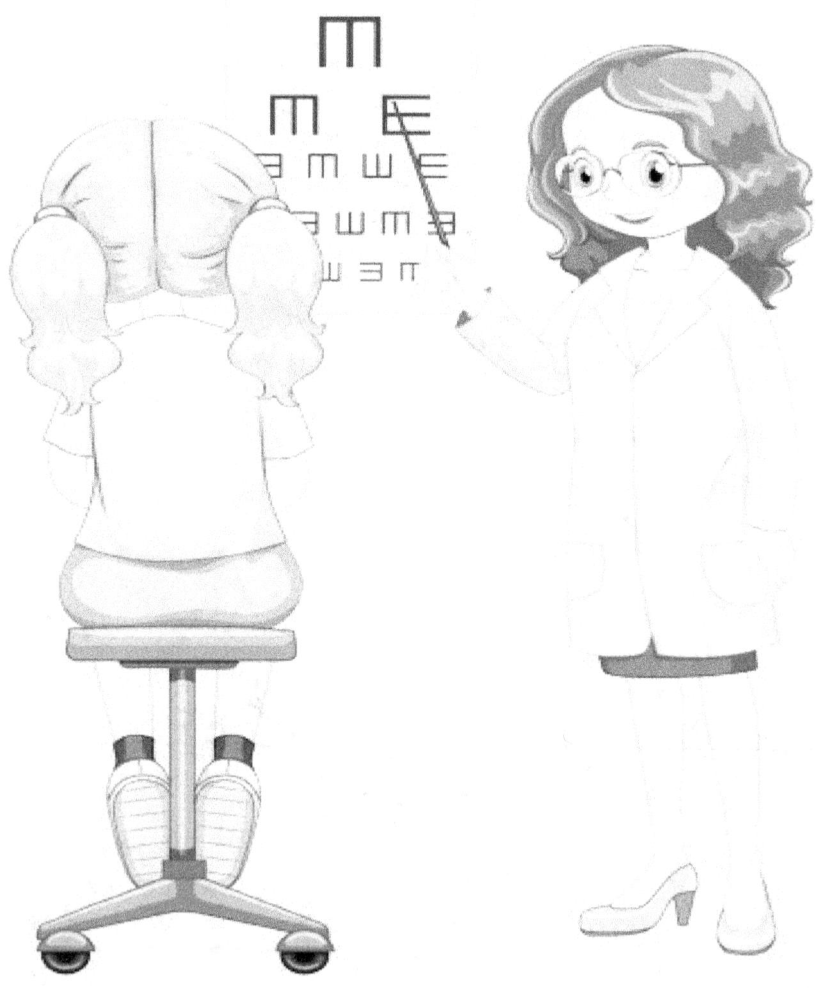

Coloring book

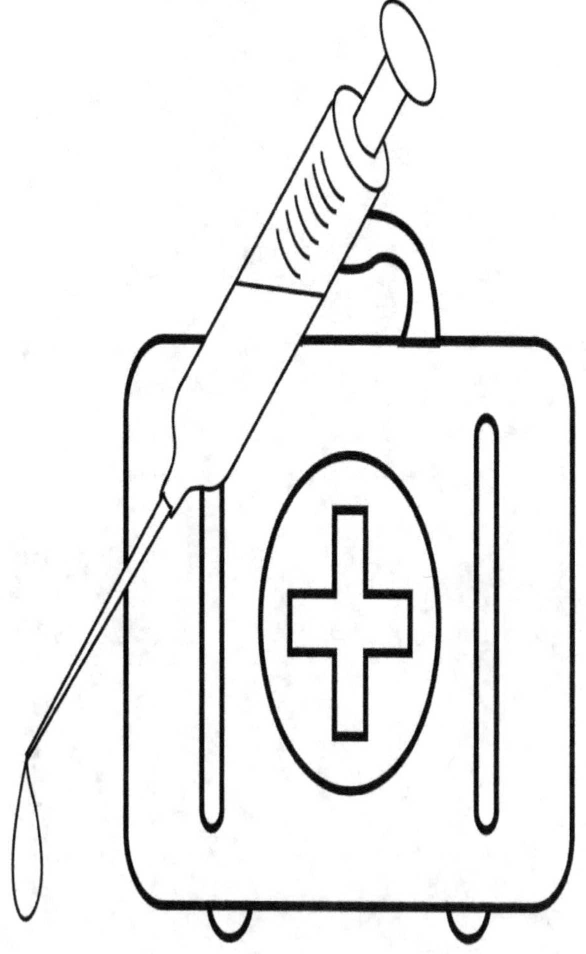

Coloring book

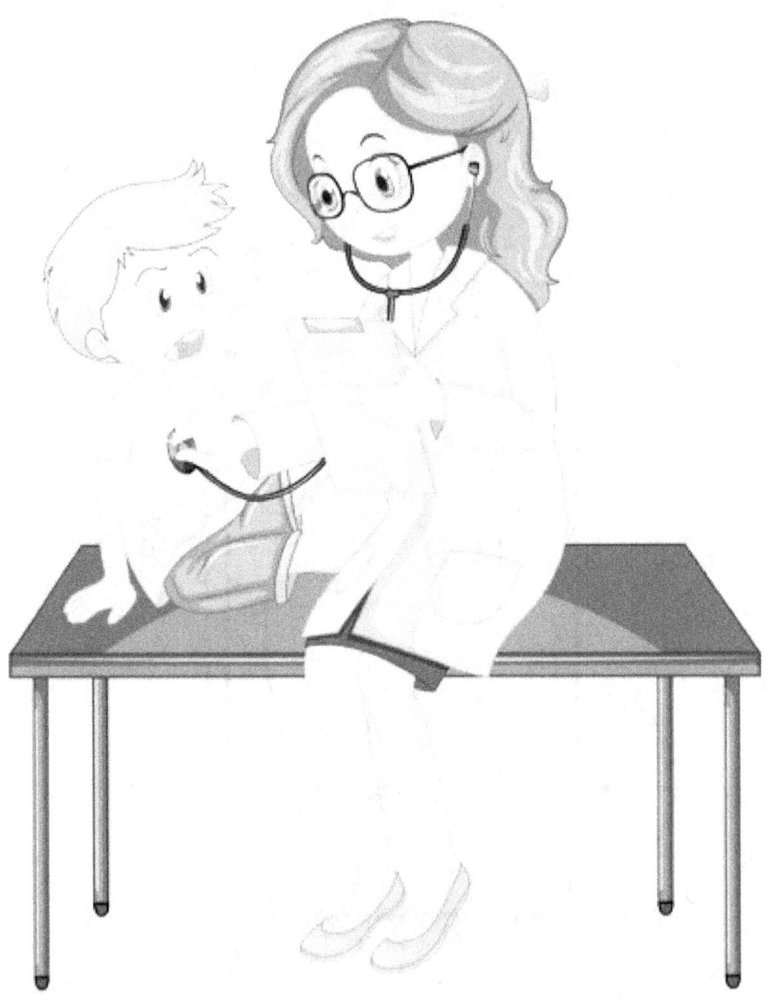

Coloring book

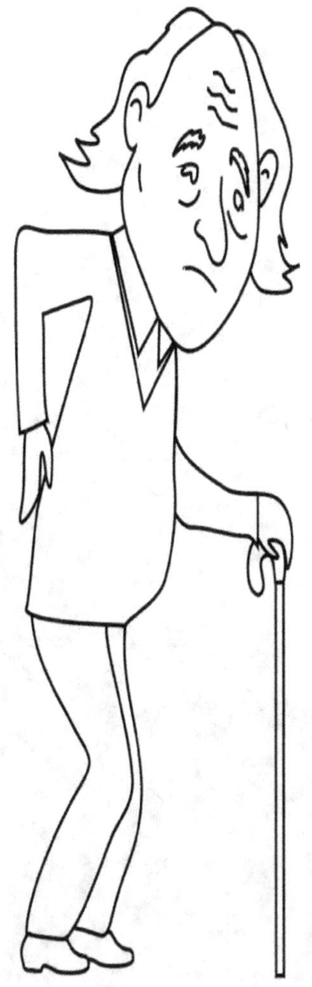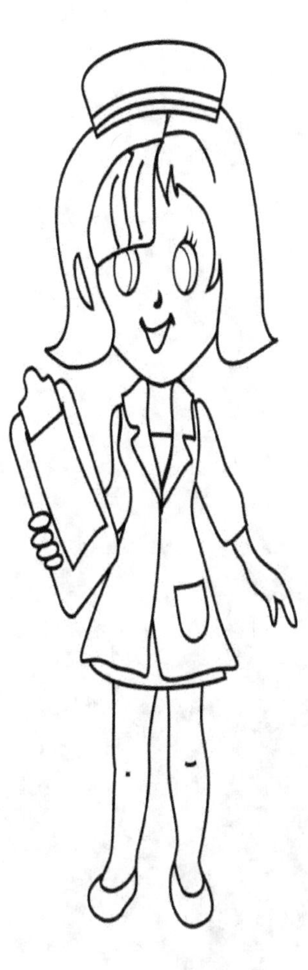

Coloring book

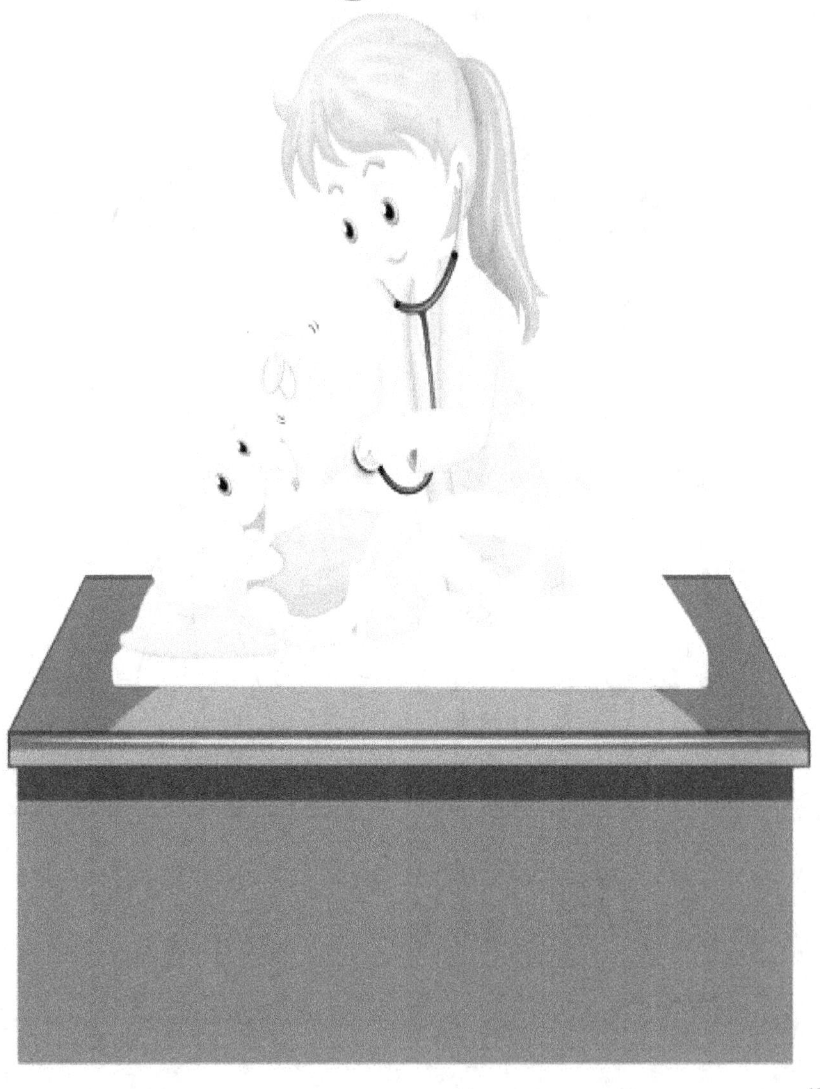

Coloring book

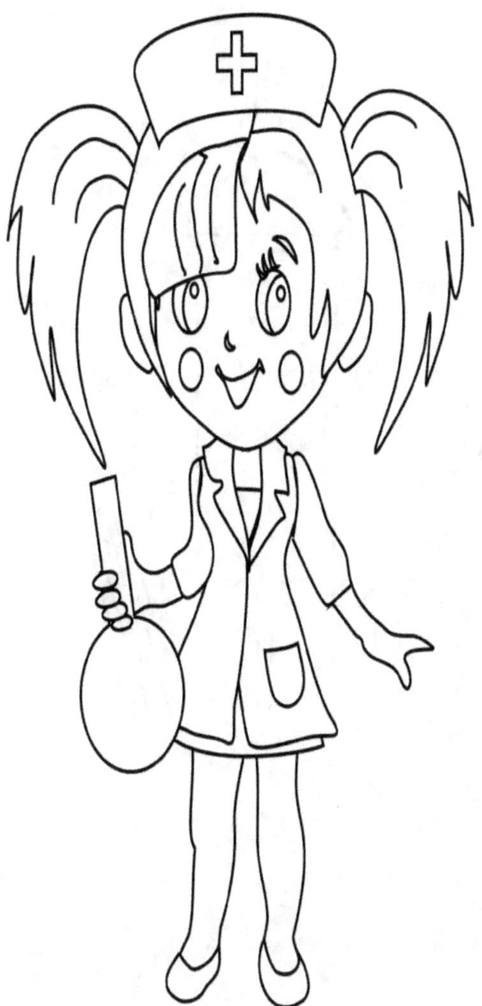

Coloring book

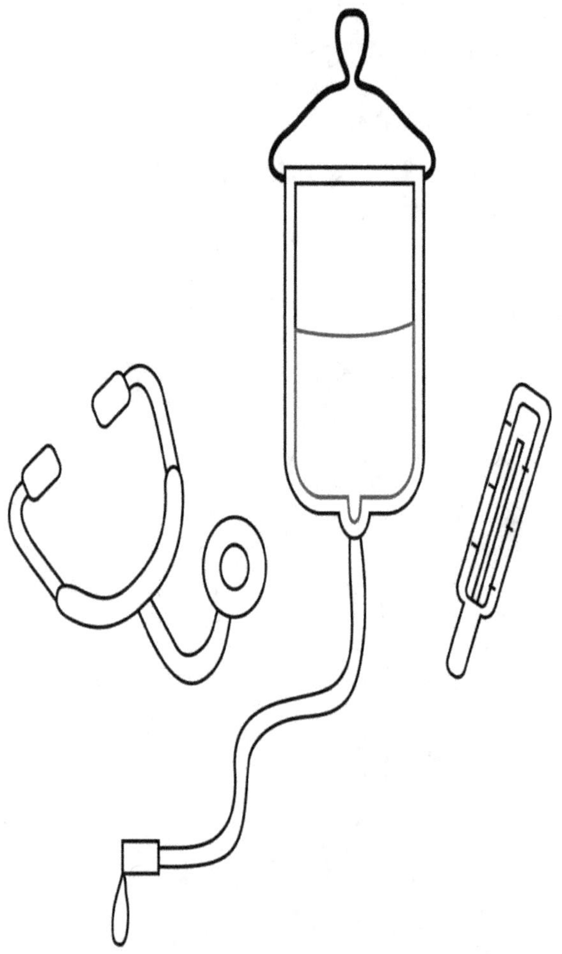

Coloring book

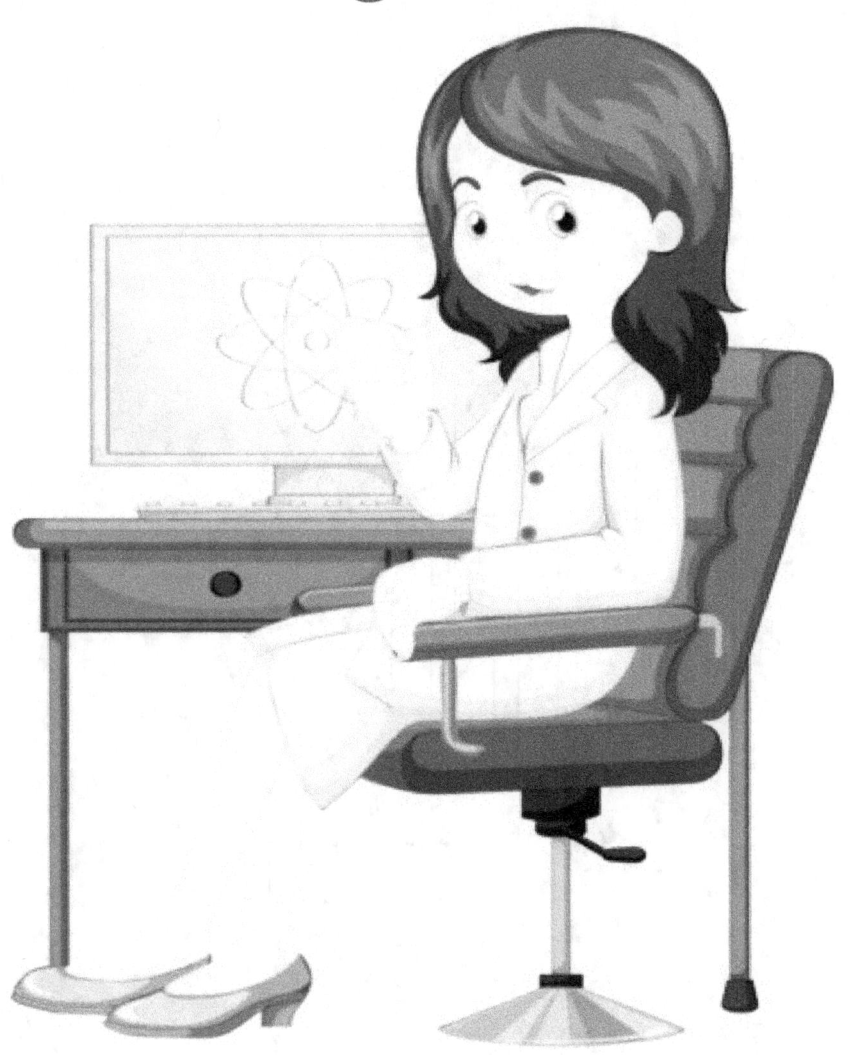

Coloring book

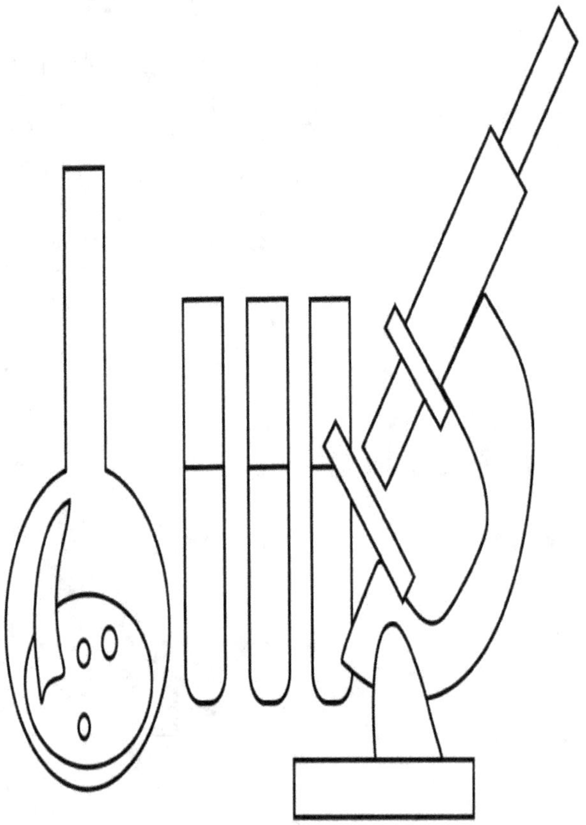

Coloring book

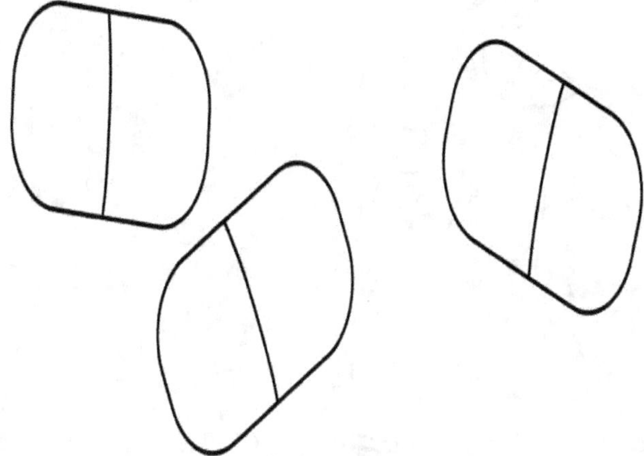

Coloring book

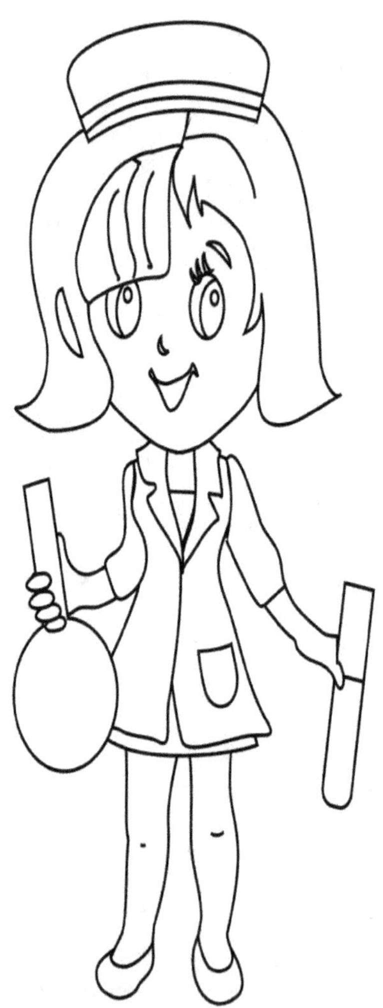

Coloring book

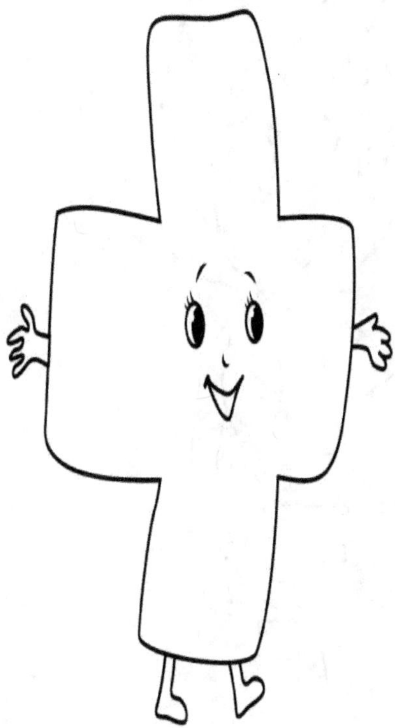

Coloring book

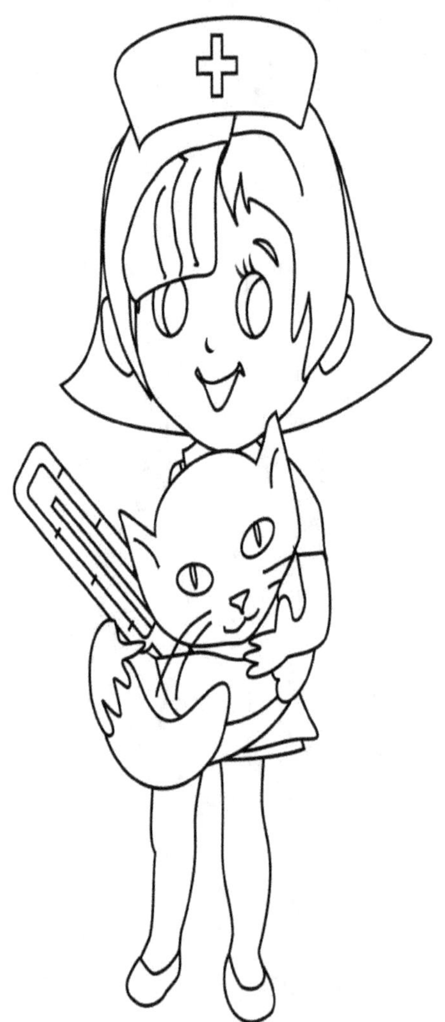

Coloring book

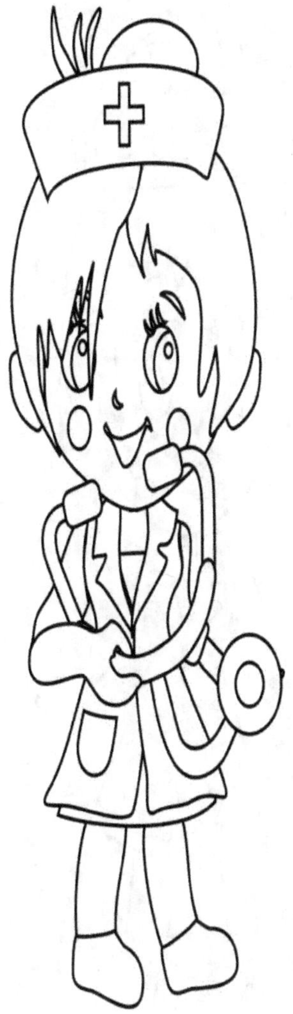

Coloring book

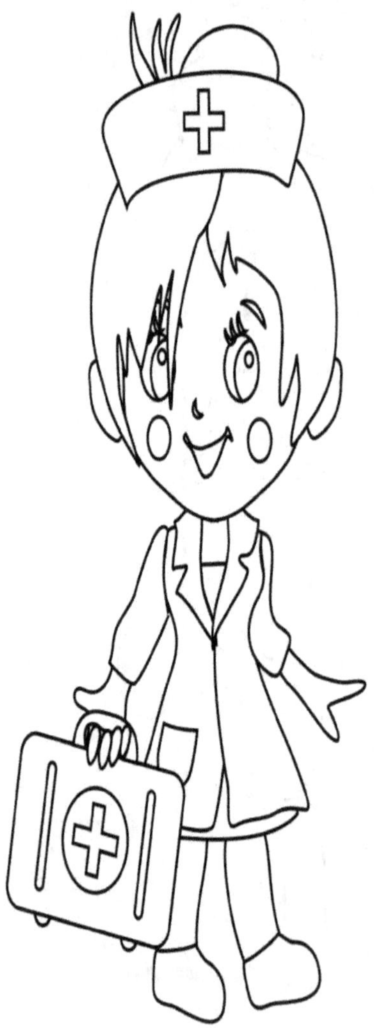

Coloring book

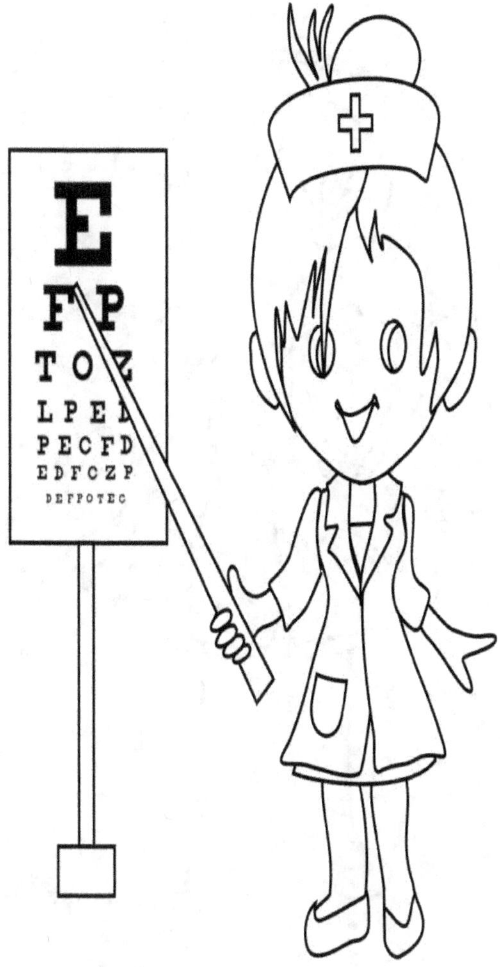

Coloring book

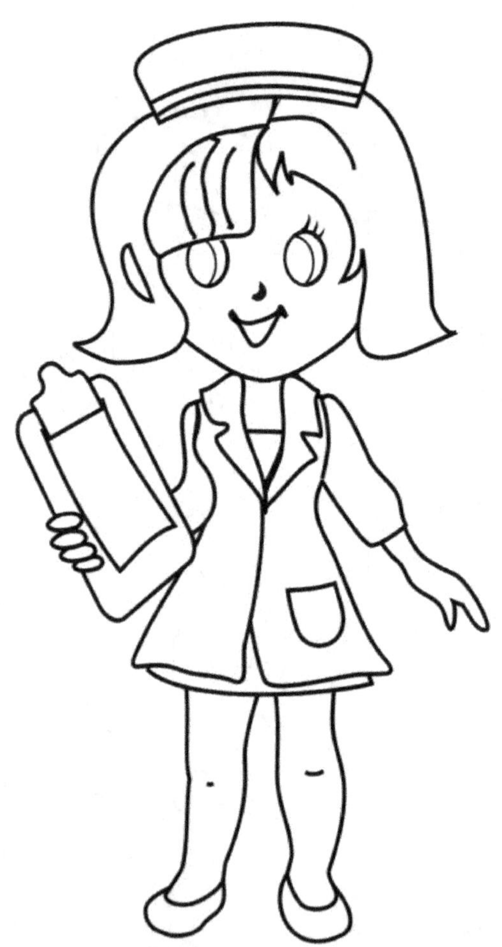

Coloring book

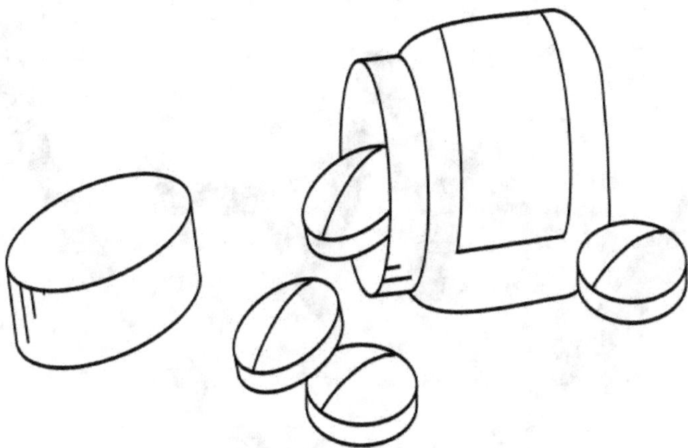

Coloring book

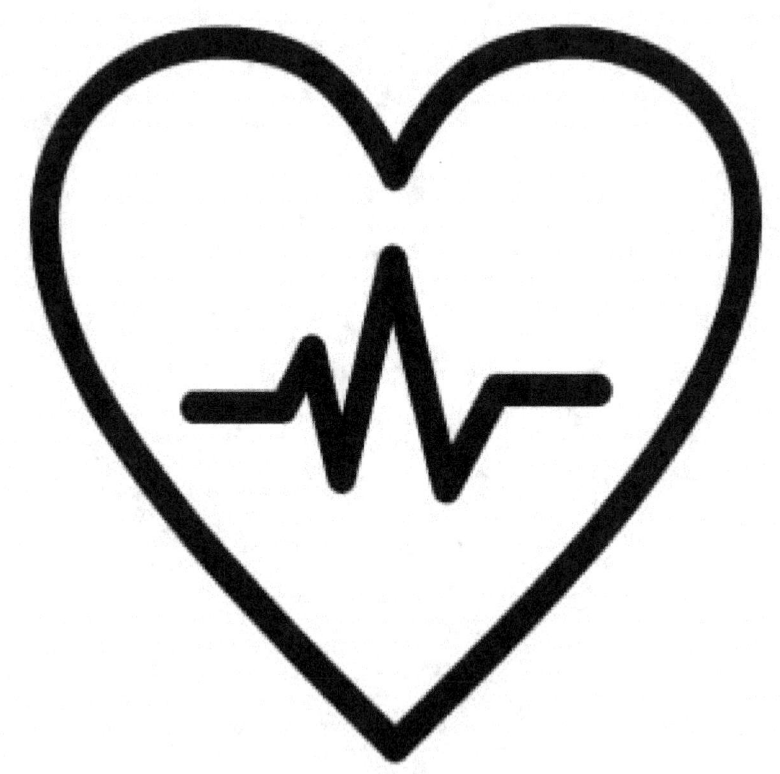

Coloring book

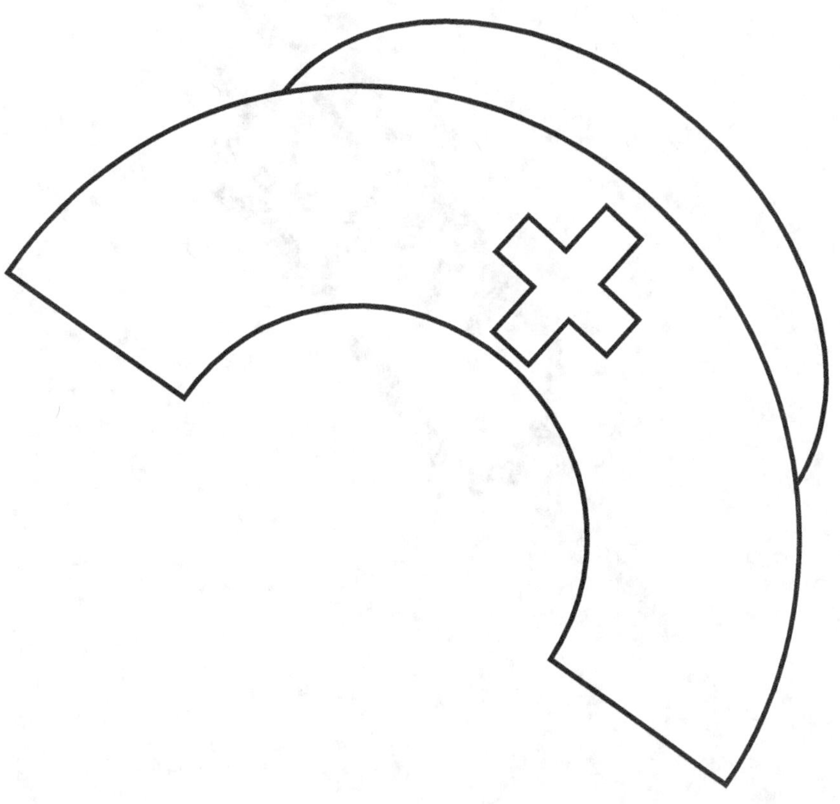

Coloring book

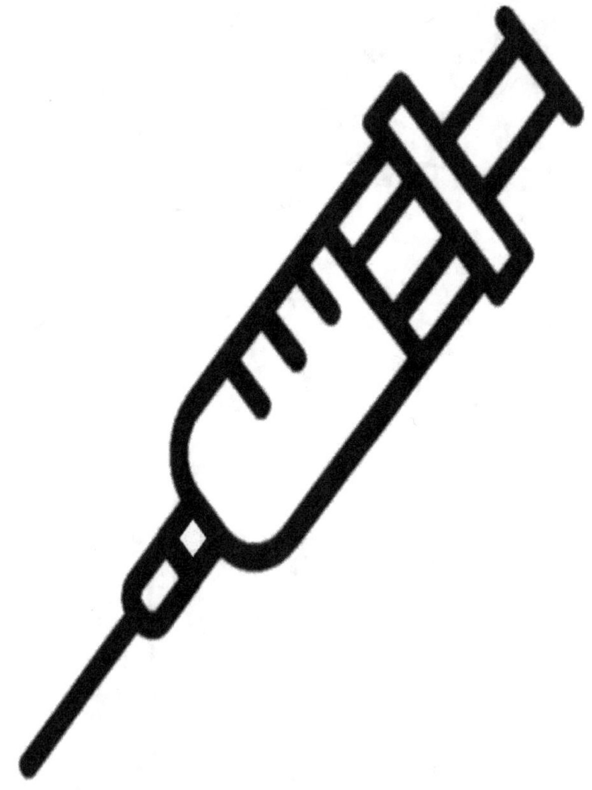

Coloring book

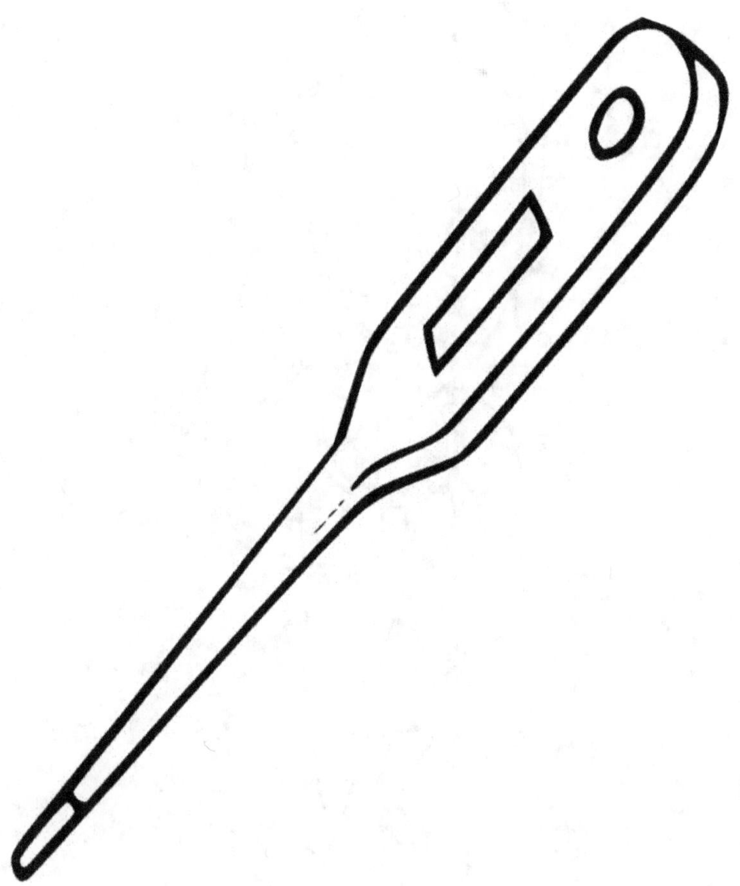

Coloring book

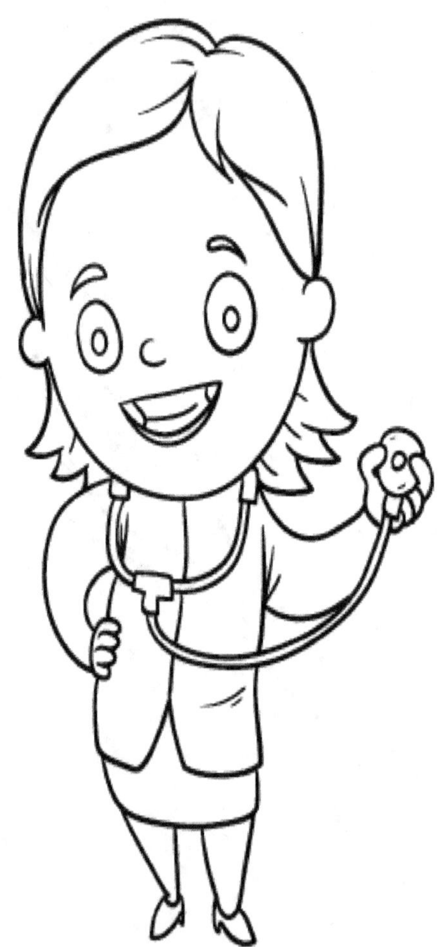

Coloring book

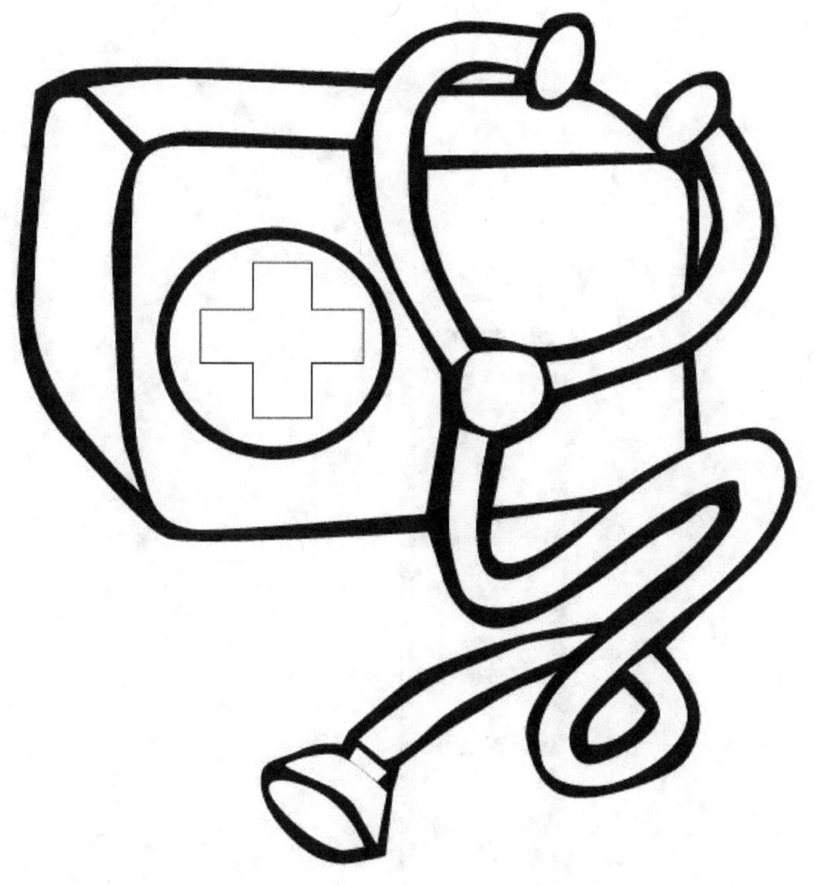

Coloring book

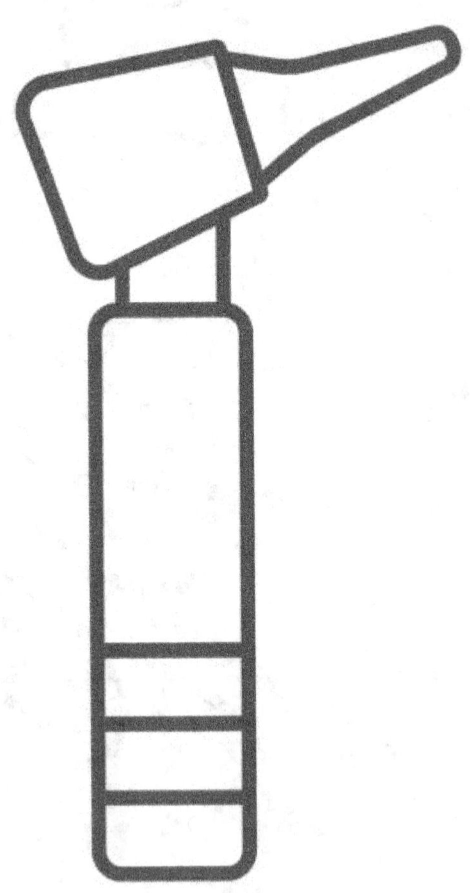

Coloring book

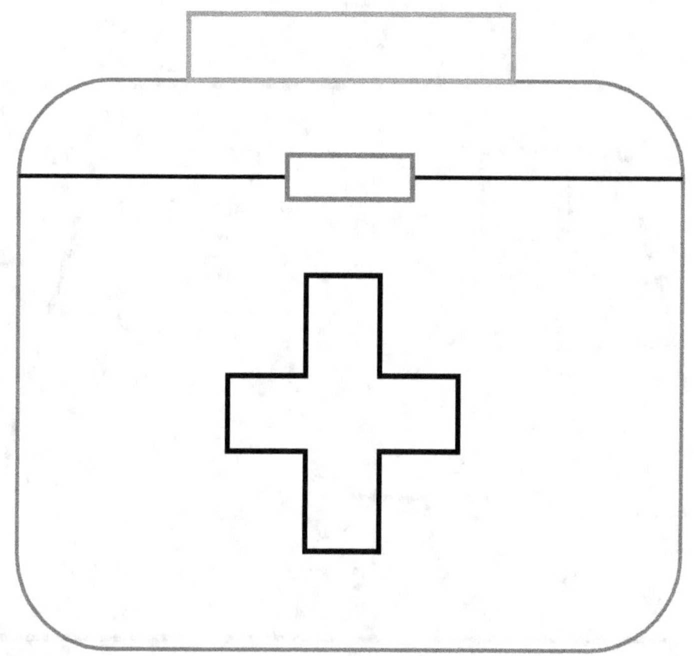

Coloring book

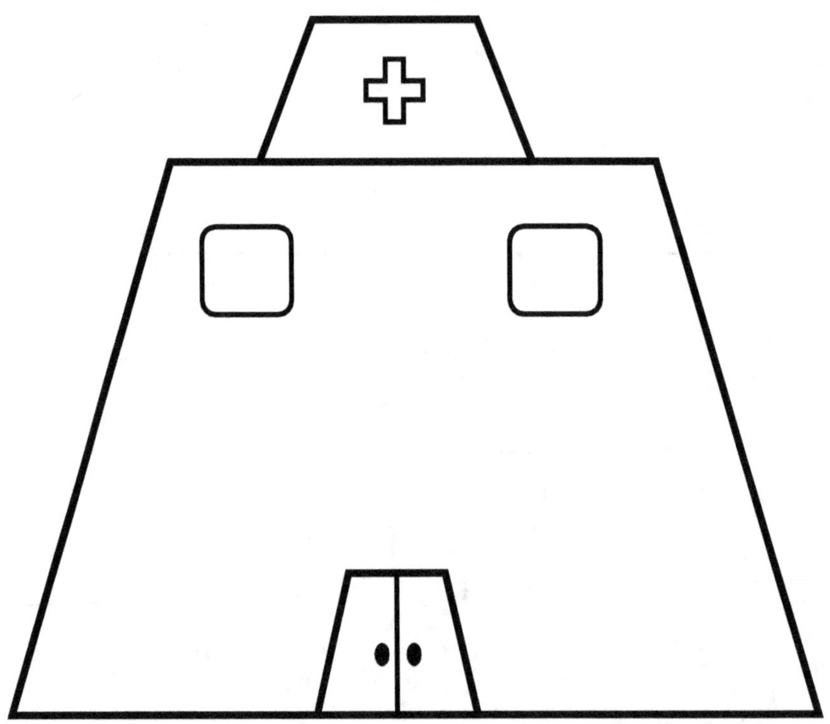

www.ingramcontent.com/pod-product-compliance
Lightning Source LLC
Chambersburg PA
CBHW050753250726
48662CB00005B/2194